TLC D

A Beginner's Overview and Review with Recipes

Table of Contents

Introduction

The path towards weight loss is often rife with a lot of misconceptions. One of these misconceptions is that losing weight can be physically demanding and exhausting. The truth, however, is that you can lose a lot of weight if you do things smartly.

The Therapeutic Lifestyle Changes Diet is a low cholesterol and low saturated fat diet that was specifically designed to assist high-risk patients lower their cholesterol levels as well as lower their risk of developing heart diseases and improve their overall health.

However, there is more to this diet than just eating the right kind of food. It will, as the name implies, require a considerable shift in paradigm on your part in order to be effective.

This guide will help you implement the TLC diet on a step-by-step basis. We will also answer some of the most frequently asked questions about it.

And, with that, we begin....

Phase 1. Know What You're Getting In To: What's the TLC Diet?

Before anything else, you should at the very least know what you are getting yourself into. What is the TLC Diet? And what can it offer to you?

To understand how a TLC diet can impact your life, it is best to learn some basic concepts revolving around the diet.

What is Cholesterol?

Cholesterol is a waxy, fat-like substance found in all cells of your body. Contrary to popular belief, not all cholesterols are bad. s In fact, your body needs cholesterol in order to make vitamin D, hormones, cell walls, and essential substances that help your body digest food.

Cholesterols cannot travel alone in the bloodstream, so they have to hitch a ride with proteins. There are two types of proteins that transport cholesterol throughout your body: high-density lipoproteins (HDL) or the "good" cholesterol and low-density lipoproteins (LDL) or the "bad" cholesterol.

Most cholesterol found in the body is LDL. They are bad in the sense that they clog the blood vessels, which will lead to disruption of the normal flow of the blood in the body. On the other hand, the HDL cholesterol removes bad cholesterol from the blood vessels and transports it back to the liver where it will be processed to be sent out to the body where it should be.

High-Blood cholesterol is a condition of having too much cholesterol from your blood. This kind of condition has no symptoms or signs. Most of the time, people do not know that their cholesterol levels are abnormally high. When there is too much cholesterol in your blood, they build up on the walls of your arteries, and will then increase your risk of developing a heart disease. Therefore, it is extremely important that you know your LDL and HDL levels, total cholesterol and triglycerides.

Unfortunately, studies have shown that one out of two Americans have high cholesterol. In 2011, 5.6 million Americans from 18 and above have high total cholesterol. As of 2010, high cholesterol levels are the primary attributor to the burden of heart disease.

Therapeutic Lifestyle Change

Invented by the National Institute of Health's National Cholesterol Education Program, and endorsed by American Heart Association as the best diet for high cholesterol patients, the Therapeutic Lifestyle Change or TLC is primarily a self-help program and regimen that can help you lower your body's cholesterol levels. It does so by cutting back on saturated fat, consuming more fiber and limiting daily cholesterol intake. This diet regimen is scientifically and statistically proven to help people manage their high cholesterol levels more effectively even without taking medication.

The Dangers of Saturated Fat

Saturated fats are fat molecules that contain double bonds between their carbon molecules because they are highly saturated with hydrogen molecules. They are usually solid at room temperature.

Eating large amounts of foods that contain high amounts of saturated fats significantly raises the level of cholesterol in your body. It has long been associated with increased susceptibility to cardiovascular diseases, stroke, obesity and even cancer.

Some of the food items that naturally contain high amounts saturated fats are the following:

- lard

- cream

- butter

- chocolate

- cheese

- processed meats

- animal fats such as beef fat (tallow) and fatty beef.

Additionally, fried foods as well as baked goods also contain extremely high levels of saturated fats.

According to the American Heart Association, a person should only achieve no more than 6% of their calories from saturated fat. This means, for example, if you need about 3,000 calories daily, no more than 180 of them should originate from saturated fats.

Phase 2. Prepare Your Pantry

The TLC Diet is all about making healthier choices, and this chapter will help you do exactly that. You need to know what to eat and what to avoid. Knowing what kind of food is good for you will ensure that your body has all the nutrients it needs.

Therefore, to get the nutrients you need, you must have a diet that is heavy on fruits, vegetables, fish, whole-grains, beans, poultry, nuts, legumes and low-fat fairy products while at the same time limiting your total consumption of sugary beverages and red meat.

The ABCs of the TLC Diet

The following are the basic elements of the TLC regimen:

- Less than 8% of your daily calories should come from saturated fats

- 25% of daily calories should come from total fat (and that includes the calories from saturated fats)

- Less than 200 mg of daily cholesterol intake

- Include 25 grams of soluble fiber a day

- Include 2 grams of plant stanols or sterols (naturally occur in grains, vegetables, fruits, nuts and seeds) a day

- Eating only enough calories to maintain a healthy Body Mass Index

- You should get at least thirty minutes of physical activity daily such as brisk walking and sports.

TLC Food Breakdown

The basic principle behind the TLC diet is to consume variety of foods that are low in saturated fats, cholesterol and trans fats but at the same time, rich in flavor. You can eat heart-healthy foods while satisfying your taste buds as well. Here is a guideline of the breakdown of TLC-approved foods (according to food groups):

- **Grains/Cereals/Breads** – They should account for six or more servings daily (you may adjust the proportion according to your daily calorie needs). This food group typically includes whole-grain cereals, bread, pasta, potatoes, rice, low-fat cookies and low-fat crackers. They are usually low in saturated fat and cholesterol while at the same time, high in fiber and complex carbohydrates.

- **Vegetables/Peas/Dry Beans** – They should account for three to five servings a day. Almost all types of vegetables are TLC-approved. You can choose from frozen, canned or fresh, but with no added sauce, salt or fat. They are extremely important in one's diet because they are the primary sources of fiber, vitamins and other nutrients that the body needs. Peas and beans are great sources of this kind of plant protein.

- **Fruits** – They should account for two to four servings daily. They are important source of nutrients, vitamins and fiber. Like the vegetable food group, almost all types of fruits are TLC-approves. They may be frozen, fresh, dried or canned but without no artificially added sugar.

- **Dairy** – They should account for two to three servings daily and should be low-fat or fat-free. They provide much more calcium than their whole milk counterparts do, but with very little amounts of saturated fat. TLC-approved dairy products include low-fat milk, fat-free milk, yogurt, buttermilk, low-fat cheese, cream cheese, sour cream, and low-fat cottage cheese.

- **Eggs** –They should account for 2 yolks per week (and that includes the yolks in baked goods and processed foods). Egg substitutes and egg whites have no cholesterol and contain lesser calories compared to whole eggs. Yolks, on the other hand, contain high amounts of dietary cholesterol. Therefore, you may eat them wholly or partially. It's your choice.

Food to Avoid

The TLC Diet can only be effective if you limit your consumption towards the recommended food groups. What kind of food, then, must you avoid at most or limit consumption to at least? These are:

- **Saturated Fats -**This can come from food like processed and red meat, chicken, eggs, whole dairy products, coconut oil, and other fatty foods.

- **Trans Fats -** This is often found in any type of food that has to be deep fried or baked in an oven. This includes french fries, donuts, cookies, and even popcorn.

- **Sugar -** Any food that is naturally sweet or artificially sweetened will be included here. That means you have to avoid ice cream, sodas, fruit drinks, pastries, and candy.

- **Salt -** Any food with a high sodium count must be avoided at all costs. This can get tricky if you are eating outside as most food prep crews will have foods seasoned beforehand. However, there is a way you can limit your exposure to salt outside (more on this later on).

- **Alcohol** - Aside from contributing to your body's eventual decline, alcohol packs a lot of calories per serving. A glass of beer contains as much as 1000 calories, whether on tap or from a bottle. This means that those that overdrink tend to go over their body's daily caloric intake limit as well.

Phase 3. Embrace the Lifestyle

The TLC Diet is more than just any kind of diet. You'll have to make some changes in the way you live and even see things in order to get the most out of the diet plan. This, in itself, will require a step-by-step process which is why it would be better if we can go through the different phases in detail.

Mental Preparation

As with every other diet, the TLC plan is a struggle between mind over matter. For the diet to work, you must make sure that the former always wins over the latter.

There are several practices that you can do to mentally prepare yourself for this diet. These include:

Making an If-Then Plan

Being strategic and analytical is one way to make the diet compatible for you. To do this, make all your decisions a set of "if-then" sequences. If you go to the grocery, then your actions will be A,B,C and so forth. If you are going to eat lunch at 11am, you are going to eat dishes A,B,C, as you have laid out in your daily meal plan (again, more on this later on).

Plotting your decisions into sets of threes at any given scenario will prevent you from falling into a deadly mental pitfall: **paralysis by analysis.**

Also, on the more practical side, it helps you become more decisive which means that you won't waste a lot of time (and money) completing your diet's objectives.

Learning from the Past

If you have failed in your past diets, don't be too hard on yourself. Look at your past failures from an objective viewpoint and try to find out exactly where you got things wrong.

Perhaps you failed in your past diet because you were overspending on your food. Or perhaps you failed because you are adding more activities without adjusting your daily nutrient intake.

This level of introspection is what will help you refine your strategies which should help you achieve the goals in your new diet plan more effectively.

Adopting a More Fluid Mindset

When it comes to diets, there is a fine distance between being committed and being stubborn or rigid. The former knows what needs to be done but is open to meeting unexpected changes in the plan. The latter, on the other hand, insists on "sticking to the plan" even if the results are not coming in the way that you want them to appear.

It is best to treat the TLC diet as a set of activities and goals, not mere rules that you have to follow to the letter. This way, you can make necessary changes to the plan to meet new demands and still lose that desired amount of weight within the set period of time.

Setting Your Expectations

What should you expect for the TLC diet to do? Here are some of its benefits.

Better Heart Health

The TLC diet is quite effective in helping the body deal with cardiovascular diseases. Since it is designed as a heart-friendly diet, the TLC plan can provide a number of benefits including lowered blood pressure, lower cholesterol levels, and reduced chances of the development of serious heart problems.

Diabetes Prevention

Research printed in the Journal of Atherosclerosis and Thrombosis would affirm that the TLC diet is effective in lowering the body's insulin levels. This is quite noticeable in cases where the person also had high cholesterol levels.

Improved Weight Loss

Although the TLC plan does not specifically deal with weight loss, it does eventually lead to there. The main goal with the TLC diet is to help the body maintain an ideal weight range and control its caloric intake.

Implementation

The TLC Diet is so straightforward that it is easy enough to follow. The main concept here is to help you lower cholesterol levels. And that goal, in itself, is not as demanding or as complicated to complete. All that is needed from you is to commit to the plan and you should see considerable progress in your body.

This simply means that you have to follow the meal plan you will set up for yourself with minimal deviations.

The TLC diet is a program that encourages you to read food labels properly. At the start, it is expected that you are going to find the scheme a bit too tedious. However, as you get used to it, you'll find yourself becoming more conscious with what you are putting in your body.

It also makes become more knowledgeable about food preparation and nutrition. Being able to calculate saturated fat percentage in every food you eat as well as portion control are just several skills you will learn with this scheme.

However, this does beg the question: *what if you can't avoid bad food entirely?*

The truth of the matter is that you can't avoid non-TLC diet compliant foods at all times. You might find yourself being treated to eat out and it would be rather odd of you to be the sole person to decline the offer. After all, you would rather not lose friends while meeting your goals.

Fortunately for you, the TLC diet was made to be flexible. This means that you can still fulfill the terms of your diet if you find yourself having to eat outside.

Pack on the Veggies

Always ask for a side of vegetables or a salad if you eat at a restaurant. If you are in a Pizzeria, always ask for extra vegetables and have the amount of cheese halved at one side.

Avoid the Fryer

Out of all the ways to prepare food, deep frying is perhaps the unhealthiest. You are better off eating food that is steam, broiled, and stir-fried. They are the lesser between nutritional evils.

Touch the Meat Last

Always eat the vegetables first, the fruits second, and the meat last. Doing so will make your stomach fuller even before you reach out for the meat. This means that your chances of eating meat are drastically reduced if you are already full from eating vegetables.

And if eating meat is not fully avoidable, choose lean meat and have it prepared in smaller portions. Also, avoid slathering your meals with a lot of sauce, gravy, or butter. These condiments contain a lot of calories and all those unwanted fats.

Recovering from Mistakes

In the battle between Mind and Matter, what if Matter won? What would you do if you actually gave in to your cravings?

The first thing to do is to STOP moping around and feeling sorry for yourself. The last thing you want to do when in a diet is to constantly beat yourself for mistakes already made. Remembering that you are not infallible tends to help you recover from your dieting mistakes faster.

The next thing that you must do is to identify where and how you made that mistake. Did you overeat when you were invited to one of your friend's Taco Tuesdays? Or was it a bowl of popcorn that did you in this time?

You have to know what food you overate the last time so you won't repeat the same mistake the next week.

And, lastly, you have to adjust your daily intake. Keep in mind that the average adult must consume no more than 2500 calories per day. Note that the recommended calorie intake for you varies depending on your height as well as your weight or weight loss targets. If you ate a lot the previous day by 500 calories, you must make adjustments to your meals on the next day so you eat no more than 2000 calories.

This is where your skill of reading food labels will come into play as you can control the amount of calories your body can take in a day.

Phase 4. Start the Day Right With These Breakfast Recipes

Breakfast is the most crucial meal of the day. This is where you get most of your nutrients to function normally until noon.

The following breakfast recipes can help lower cholesterol by capping unhealthy fats that raise your body's total bad cholesterol levels and at the same time, cleanse your digestive system of cholesterols. These dishes contain powerful cholesterol-fighting ingredients that are not only heart-healthy, but extremely delicious as well.

Caramelized Onion, Parmesan Cheese and Arugula Omelet

Preparation Time: 30 minutes

Cooking Time: 20 minutes

Yield: 2 servings (1/2 omelet each plate)

Calories: 116

Ingredients:

- 1 tablespoon of extra-virgin olive oil

- Cooking spray (preferably PAM® Olive Oil No-Stick Cooking Spray)

- 1 teaspoon of no-cholesterol butter (preferably Fleischmann's® Original-stick)

- ¼ cup of arugula

- 2 pieces of thinly sliced, medium-sized onions (halved)

- ¼ teaspoon of ground black pepper

- ¾ cup of Egg Beaters Original

- 2 teaspoons of balsamic vinegar

- ¼ cup of shredded Parmesan cheese

Instructions:

1. Melt the butter and oil in a pan over medium-low heat.

2. When the butter has melted, add the onions. Gently stir to coat. Continue stirring for ten minutes while stirring occasionally. When the onions have softened and turned translucent in color, you may add the vinegar.

3. Cook the onions and vinegar mixture for another 20 minutes. Reserve 1/3 cup of the mixture for later use. Store the reserved mixture in an airtight container.

4. To make the omelet, spray a skillet with the cooking spray and heat it over medium-high heat. Cook the reserved onions, garlic, and arugula into the preheated skillet. Continue sautéing them until the arugula has wilted (approximately one minute).

5. In a bowl, combine the cheese, pepper and Egg Beaters. Mix the mixture thoroughly. Pour them in a skillet.

6. Wait until the edges are set before pulling the edges towards the center. Repeat. Continue cooking until the center is set (approximately 2 minutes). Fold and cut the omelet in half. Serve immediately.

Black Beans and Quinoa

Preparation Time: 15 minutes

Cooking Time: 35 minutes

Ingredients:

- 1 teaspoon of vegetable oil
- ½ cup of chopped fresh cilantro
- 1 piece of chopped onion
- 2 cans of rinsed and drained black beans (15-ounces can)
- 3 cloves of chopped garlic
- 1 cup of corn kernels (frozen)
- ¾ cup of quinoa
- Salt and ground black pepper (to taste)
- 1 ½ cup of vegetable broth
- ¼ teaspoon of cayenne pepper
- 1 teaspoon of ground cumin

Instructions:

1. Sauté onion and garlic in a saucepan over medium heat for ten minutes.

2. Add quinoa to the onion and garlic mixture. Cover the spices with vegetable broth.

3. Season the mixture with salt, pepper, cumin and cayenne pepper. Boil and cover. Let it simmer for 20 minutes.

4. Stir in corn into the saucepan and continue to simmer for five more minutes.

5. Afterwards, stir in the cilantro and black beans.

Potato-Parmesan Pancakes

Preparation Time: 10 minutes

Cooking Time: 12 minutes

Yield: 4 servings (2 pancakes each plate)

Calories: 150

Ingredients:

- 2 cups of mashed potatoes
- ¼ cup of divided breadcrumbs (seasoned)
- 2 tablespoons of finely chopped green onions
- 2 tablespoons of freshly grated Parmesan cheese)

- 1 egg white (large)
- 2 tablespoons of divided olive oil

Instructions:

1. In a big bowl, combine chives, potatoes, egg white and two tablespoons of bread crumbs.

2. On a clean plate, combine cheese and two tablespoons of breadcrumbs.

3. Divide the earlier potato mixture into eight equal portions and roll them in the breadcrumb mixture while shaping each portion into a patty (1/4-inch thick).

4. Heat one teaspoon of olive oil in a nonstick skillet. Cook four patties in the preheated pan for four minutes on each side. Repeat with one teaspoon of oil for the remaining patties.

5. Serve the pancakes with low-fat sour cream and applesauce.

Low-Cholesterol Waldorf Salad

Preparation Time: 15 minutes

Cooking Time: 35 minutes

Yield: 3 servings (1 cup)

Calories: 93 calories

Ingredients:

- ½ cup of raisins
- 2 tablespoons of apple-flavored yoghurt (fat-free)
- ½ cup of apple juice
- 2 tablespoons of mayonnaise (fat-free)
- 1 cup of finely chopped celery
- ¼ cup of toasted walnuts (coarsely chopped)
- 1 cup of Granny Smith apple (chopped)

Instructions:

1. Combine apple juice and raisins in a bowl (microwave-safe) and microwave on high heat for thirty seconds.

2. Let it stand for two minutes. Drain.

3. Combine celery, apple, walnuts, and raisins in a bowl. Stir in the yoghurt and mayonnaise into the mixture. Serve immediately.

Breakfast Muffins

Preparation Time: 15 minutes

Cooking Time: 35 minutes

Yield: 18 servings

Calories: 186

Ingredients:

- Cooking spray
- 1 cup of fat-free yoghurt (plain)
- 1 cup of whole wheat flour
- 1 cup of mashed banana (ripe)
- 1 cup of regular oats
- 1 egg (large)
- ¾ cup of packed brown sugar
- 1 cup of chopped dates (pitted)
- 1 tablespoon of wheat bran
- ¾ cup of finely chopped walnuts
- 2 tablespoons of baking soda
- ½ cup of dried pineapple (chopped)
- ¼ teaspoon of salt
- 3 tablespoons of ground flaxseed

Instructions:

1. Preheat the oven until it reaches the temperature of 350 degrees F. Place liners in all of the muffin cups and coat them with cooking spray.

2. Spoon flour into a measuring cup. Use a knife to level the flour.

3. Combine the flour, oats, sugar, wheat bran, baking soda and salt in a large bowl.

4. Combine them thoroughly.

5. Make a well at the center of the mixture.

6. On the other hand, combine banana, egg, and yoghurt in a small bowl and add to the earlier flour mixture.

7. Mix well. Fold in pineapple, walnuts and dates into the mixture.

8. Spoon batter into the lined muffin cups. Sprinkle the top with flax seed. Bake the muffins at 350 degrees F for 20 minutes.

9. Remove the muffins from the pans. Let them cool on a wire rack.

Low Cholesterol Apple-Cinnamon Granola Breakfast

Preparation Time: 15 minutes

Cooking Time: 40 minutes

Yield: 6 servings

Calories: 116

Ingredients:

- 3 cups of regular oats
- 2 tablespoons of butter
- 1 cup of whole-grain oat cereal (preferably Cheerios)
- 1/3 cup of applesauce
- 1/3 cup of oat bran
- ¼ cup of honey
- 1/3 cup of finely chopped walnuts
- 2 tablespoons of brown sugar
- 2 teaspoons of ground cinnamon
- 1 cup of finely chopped dried apple
- ¼ teaspoon of ground cardamom

Instructions:

1. Preheat the oven until it reaches the temperature of 250 degrees F.

2. Combine regular oats, oat cereal, oat bran, walnuts, cinnamon, and cardamom in a large bowl.

3. Stir well to combine the ingredients thoroughly.

4. Melt two tablespoons of butter in a saucepan over medium heat. Add honey, brown sugar and 1/3 cup of applesauce into the heated saucepan. Boil.

5. Cook the mixture for a minute. Pour applesauce mixture on top of the oat mixture while stirring well to coat. Spread the resulting mixture in a jellyroll pan.

6. Make sure to coat the jellyroll pan with cooking spray. Bake the mixture at 250 degrees F for 1 ½ hours while stirring frequently every thirty minutes. Let it cool.

7. Stir in finely chopped apples into the granola. Store them in an airtight container.

Classic Buttermilk Pancakes

Preparation Time: 15 minutes

Cooking Time: 35 minutes

Yield: 12 servings

Calories: 104

Ingredients:

- 1 cup of all-purpose flour
- 1 cup of buttermilk
- 3 tablespoons of sugar
- ¼ cup of canola oil
- ½ teaspoon of baking powder
- 1 teaspoon of vanilla extract
- ½ teaspoon of baking soda
- 3 egg whites

Instructions:

1. Combine all-purpose flour, sugar, baking powder and baking soda in a small bowl.

2. In another bowl, combine vanilla, oil and butter milk. Mix them thoroughly before adding the second mixture to the first.

3. In another bowl, beat the egg whites until they form small peaks. Fold them into batter.

4. Pour batter into a hot griddle (coated with cooking spray). Cook until both sides are lightly browned. Serve with maple syrup on top.

Spinach, Feta, and Tomato Omelet

Preparation Time: 15 minutes

Cooking Time: 15 minutes

Yield: 1 serving

Calories: 150

Ingredients:

- Cooking spray
- ¼ cup of Roma tomatoes (chopped)
- ¾ cup of Egg Beaters Liquid Egg Whites
- 2 tablespoons of crumbled feta cheese (fat reduced)
- 1/8 teaspoon of ground black pepper
- ¼ cup of baby spinach leaves (chopped)

Instructions:

1. Spray small amounts of cooking spray in a nonstick skillet. Heat them over medium heat until hot.

2. Cook the Egg Beaters in the heated skillet. Season Egg Beaters with pepper. Cook for two minutes.

3. Lift the edges to cook the other side of the egg. Cook for three more minutes.

4. Top the half of the omelet with tomatoes, spinach and feta cheese. Fold the other half of the omelet over the filling. Serve.

Ten-Minute Pasta Toss

Preparation Time: 20 minutes

Cooking Time: 10 minutes

Yield: 8 servings

Calories: 150

Ingredients:

- 16 ounces of rotini pasta
- 1 ¼ teaspoons of garlic powder
- 4 tablespoons of olive oil
- 1 ¼ teaspoons of dried basil
- 4 pieces of chicken breast halves (boneless and skinless)
- 1 ¼ teaspoons of dried oregano
- 3 cloves of minced garlic
- 1 cup of finely chopped sun-dried tomatoes
- 1 ¼ teaspoons of salt
- ¼ cup of finely grated Parmesan cheese

Instructions:

1. Boil a large pot of salted water. Cook the rotini pasta into the boiling water for about eight minutes. Drain.

2. Sauté chicken, salt, garlic, garlic powder, oregano and basil in a preheated pot over medium-high heat for about ten minutes.

3. Add the tomatoes and cook for two minutes. Remove from heat. Pour the cooked rotini pasta into the pot with sauce and toss until well combined.

4. Serve with Parmesan cheese on top.

Low-Cholesterol Swiss Asparagus Omelet

Preparation Time: 20 minutes

Cooking Time: 10 minutes

Yield: 1 serving

Calories: 194

Ingredients:

- Cooking spray
- 5 pieces of trimmed and cooked asparagus spears
- ¾ cup of Egg Beaters Liquid Egg Whites
- 1 slice of halved Swiss cheese (fat-reduced)
- 1/8 teaspoon of ground black pepper

Instructions:

1. Spray small amounts of cooking spray in a nonstick skillet and heat it over medium heat until hot. Add the Egg Beaters and cook for two minutes until the eggs begin to set.

2. Lift the edges to cook the other side of the egg. Cook for three more minutes.

3. Top the half of the omelet with pepper, feta cheese and asparagus. Fold the other half of the omelet over the filling. Serve.

Phase 5. Master The TLC Way With These Main Dish Recipes

Your Lunch and Dinner could also benefit from a revamp. Lunch is especially crucial as this gives you the nutrients you need for the next few hours. Here are some recipes to consider so you can follow your TLC diet all day long.

Orecchiette with Chickpeas and Broccoli Rabe

Preparation Time: 20 minutes

Cooking Time: 10 minutes

Yield: 1 serving

Calories: 194

Ingredients:

- 4 ounces of whole wheat Orecchiette

- 4 cloves of garlic (minced)

- ¼ teaspoon of freshly ground pepper

- ½ bunch of trimmed broccoli rabe (cut into 2-inch pieces)

- ½ teaspoon of minced rosemary (fresh)

- ¾ cup of vegetarian broth (chicken-flavored)

- 1 can of drained and rinsed chickpeas (8-ounce)

- 2 teaspoons of all-purpose flour

- 2 teaspoons of red wine vinegar

- 1 tablespoon of extra-virgin olive oil

Instructions:

1. Boil a large saucepan of salted water. Cook pasta in the salted water for six minutes.

2. Add broccoli rabe into the pot while stirring occasionally. Cook the pasta and broccoli rabe for another three minutes before draining. Dry the pot.

3. Whisk flour and broth in a small bowl.

4. Sauté garlic and rosemary in a preheated pan over medium-high heat. Stir constantly for one minute. Whisk in the broth mixture and simmer. Stir constantly. Add vinegar, chickpeas, pepper, salt and the pasta mixture. Cook for two more minutes while stirring constantly.

5. Serve.

Lemon and Almond Crusted Fish with Spinach

Preparation Time: 24 minutes

Cooking Time: 10 minutes

Yield: 4 servings

Calories: 249

Ingredients:

- Juice and zest of one lemon (divided)
- 1 teaspoon of kosher salt
- ½ cup of coarsely chopped almonds
- Freshly ground pepper (to taste)
- 1 tablespoon of fresh dill (finely chopped)
- 1 ¼ pounds of halibut (cut into four equal portions)
- 1 tablespoon of olive oil (extra-virgin)
- 4 teaspoons of Dijon mustard
- Lemon wedges (garnish)
- 2 teaspoons of olive oil (extra-virgin)
- 1 pound of baby spinach

Instructions:

Preheat the oven until it reaches the temperature of 400 degrees F.

Spray small amounts of cooking spray in a rimmed baking sheet.

Combine almonds, lemon zest, fill, pepper, ½ teaspoon of salt and 1 teaspoon of oil in a small bowl.

Place the four portions of fish on the oiled baking sheet and spread each portion with a teaspoon of mustard.

Divide the almond mixture into four equal portions while pressing it onto the mustard. Bake the fish for nine minutes or more (depending on the thickness). Make sure that the fish is opaque in the center before removing it from the oven.

Meanwhile, heat two teaspoons of oil in a Dutch over medium-high heat. Sauté garlic for about 30 seconds in the preheated oven. Stir in lemon juice, spinach and the remaining salt. Season it with pepper. Stir well for four minutes. Cover

Serve the fish with lemon wedges and spinach on the sides. Enjoy!

Tomato and Turkey Panini

Preparation Time: 10 minutes

Cooking Time: 25 minutes

Yield: 4 servings

Calories: 249

Ingredients:

- 3 tablespoons of mayonnaise (fat-reduced)
- 1 teaspoon of lemon juice
- 2 tablespoons of plain yoghurt (non-fat)
- Freshly ground pepper (to taste)
- 2 tablespoons of shredded Parmesan cheese
- 8 slices of thinly sliced turkey (sodium-reduced)
- 2 tablespoons of finely chopped fresh basil
- 8 slices of tomato
- 2 teaspoons of canola oil

Instructions:

1. Combine Parmesan, mayonnaise, yoghurt, lemon juice, basil and pepper in a bowl.

Spread two teaspoons of the mixture on each bread.

2. Divide tomato and turkey slices evenly among the four slices of bread. Top each with the remaining bread.

3. Meanwhile, heat one teaspoon of oil in a skillet over medium heat. Place two panini in the pan. Place the skillet on top of the panini. Use the cans to weigh it down. Cook the panini until they turn golden on one side (which will take about two minutes.)

4. Reduce the heat to low. Flow the Panini. Repeat the same process on the other side. Cook the remaining Panini. Serve immediately.

Penne with Asparagus and Chicken

Preparation Time: 15 minutes

Cooking Time: 20 minutes

Yield: 8 servings

Calories: 332

Ingredients:

- 1 package of dried penne pasta

- ½ cup of chicken broth (low sodium)

- 5 tablespoons of divided olive oil

- 1 bunch of trimmed slender asparagus spears

- 2 pieces of cubed breast halves (skinless and boneless)

- 1 clove of thinly sliced garlic

- Salt and pepper (to taste)

- ¼ cup of Parmesan cheese

- Garlic powder

Instructions:

1. Boil a large pot of salted water. Add pasta and cook for 10 minutes. Drain. Set aside for later use.

2. Warm three tablespoons of olive oil in a skillet over medium-high heat. Add chicken into the preheated skillet. Season it with pepper, salt and garlic powder. Cook for five minutes. Make sure that the chicken is thoroughly browned before transferring the chicken to paper towels.

3. Pour the chicken broth into the skillet and add the asparagus, garlic, salt, pepper and a pinch of garlic powder. Cover. Steam the mixture for ten minutes.

4. Return the cooked chicken into the skillet. Pour the chicken mixture into the cooked pasta and mix well. Let it sit for five minutes.

5. Drizzle with 2 tablespoon of olive oil and sprinkle with Parmesan cheese on top. Serve.

Black Beans and Rice

Preparation Time: 5 minutes

Cooking Time: 25 minutes

Yield: 8 servings

Calories: 140

Ingredients:

- 1 teaspoon of olive oil
- 1 ½ cups of vegetable broth (low sodium)
- 1 chopped onion
- 1 teaspoon of ground cumin
- 1 cloves of minced garlic
- ¼ teaspoon of cayenne pepper
- ¾ cup of uncooked white rice
- 3 ½ cups of drained black beans in can

Instructions:

1. Heat the olive oil in a stockpot over medium heat. Sauté the onion and garlic in the heated stockpot for four minutes. Add the rice and cook for another two minutes.

2. Add the vegetable broth. Boil. Lower the heat and cook for 20 minutes. Add the black beans and the spices on the list. Serve while hot.

Slow-Cooked Pulled Pork BBQ

Preparation Time: 15 minutes

Cooking Time: 7 hours and 10 minutes

Yield: 8 servings

Calories: 335

Ingredients:

- 2 pounds of pork tenderloin
- 8 pieces of split and toasted hamburger buns
- 1 can of root beer
- 1 bottle of barbecue sauce

Instructions:

1. Place the pork in a slow cooker. Pour the beer on top the meat. Cover. Cook on low for seven hours.

2. Drain well.

3. Stir in barbecue sauce. Serve on top of the buns.

Chickpea Curry

Preparation Time: 15 minutes

Cooking Time: 15 minutes

Yield: 8 servings

Calories: 254

Ingredients:

- 2 tablespoons of vegetable oil
- 1 cup of finely chopped fresh cilantro
- 2 minced onions
- 2 cans of garbanzo beans (15-ounce)
- 2 cloves of minced garlic
- 1 teaspoon of ground turmeric
- 2 teaspoons of finely chopped ginger root (fresh)
- 1 teaspoon of cayenne pepper
- 6 whole cloves
- salt
- 2 crushed cinnamon sticks
- 1 teaspoon of ground coriander
- 1 teaspoon of ground cumin

Instructions:

1. Heat oil in a frying pan over medium heat.

2. Sauté onion until they turn tender. Stir in ginger, garlic, coriander, cinnamon, cumin, cayenne and turmeric. Cook them for one minute while stirring constantly.

3. Mix in garbanzo beans and its liquid into the mixture. Continue cooking while stirring frequently to make sure that the ingredients are well blended and heated. Remove from heat.

4. Stir in cilantro. Serve.

Slow-Cooked Honeyed Garlic Chicken

Preparation Time: 25 minutes

Cooking Time: 4 hours and 15 minutes

Yield: 8 servings

Calories: 254

Ingredients:

- 1 tablespoon of vegetable oil
- ¼ cup of water
- 10 pieces of chicken thighs (boneless and skinless)
- 2 tablespoons of cornstarch
- ¾ cup of honey
- 1 can of drained pineapple tidbits (juice reserved)
- ¾ cup of lite soy sauce
- 1 tablespoon of fresh ginger root (minced)
- 3 tablespoons of ketchup
- 2 cloves of crushed garlic

Instructions:

1. Heat oil in a medium-sized skillet over medium heat. Cook the chicken thighs in the

preheated skillet until they turn evenly brown on all sides. Transfer the chicken thighs in a slow cooker.

2. In a bowl, mix soy sauce, honey, garlic, ginger, ketchup, and the reserved pineapple juice. Pour the mixture into the slow cooker with the chicken. Cover. Cook for four hours on high.

3. Mix water and cornstarch in a bowl. Remove thighs from the slow cooker. Blend the cornstarch and water mixture into the sauce in the slow-cooker. Return the chicken into the slow cooker. Add the pineapple tidbits.

4. Serve immediately.

Step 6. Sweeten Things Up: Make Your New Lifestyle Sustainable

One common misconception that we would like to debunk is that sweets are off-limits. Just because you want to have a more heart-healthy lifestyle that does not mean you have to forsake your sweets. You just have to be a bit more careful and creative when choosing the ingredients of your desert.

Common dessert ingredients that have high fat content such as whipped cream and butter contain high levels of saturated fat that increases cholesterol levels in the body. As discussed in the earlier chapters, high cholesterol can lead to stroke, kidney problems and heart attacks. The following desserts contain low saturated fat:

Low-Cholesterol Pretzel Turtles

Preparation Time: 10 minutes

Cooking Time: 4 minutes

Yield: 20 servings

Ingredients:

- 20 pieces of small pretzels

- 20 pieces of chocolate covered caramel-flavored candies

- 20 pieces of pecan halves

Instructions:

1. Preheat the oven until it reaches the desired temperature of 300 degrees F.

2. Place the pretzels in a parchment-lined cookie sheet. Put one candy on each pretzel.

3. Cook them in the oven for four minutes. While the candy is still warm, put a pecan half on each pretzel. Let them cool down before transferring them in an airtight container.

Low-Cholesterol Strawberry Shortcakes

Preparation Time: 10 minutes

Cooking Time: 4 minutes

Yield: 6 servings

Calories: 113

Ingredients:

- 1 tablespoon of calorie-free sweetener
- ¼ teaspoon of almond extract
- 1 tablespoon of cornstarch
- 1 ½ cups of fresh strawberries (sliced)
- 1 cup of orange juice
- 6 pieces of sponge cake dessert shells

Instructions:

1. In a small saucepan, combine cornstarch and sweetener. Add orange juice into the mixture and boil.

2. Stir constantly for one minute. Remove from heat. Add in extract. Let it cool down.

3. Combine strawberries and orange juice mixture in a big bowl. Stir frequently. Cover. Refrigerate for 30 minutes. To serve, pour the sauce into the dessert shells.

Traditional Cream Cheese Brownies

Preparation Time: 20 minutes

Cooking Time: 40 minutes

Yield: 16 servings

Calories: 127

Ingredients:

- ¾ cup of sugar
- ½ cup of all-purpose flour
- ¼ cup and 2 tablespoons of softened stick margarine (calorie-reduced)
- ¼ cup of unsweetened cocoa
- 1 large egg
- Cooking spray
- 1 large egg white
- 1 piece of softened cream cheese (8-ounce block)
- 1 tablespoon of vanilla extract
- ¼ cup of calorie-free sweetener
- 3 tablespoons of low-fat milk (1%)

Instructions:

1. Preheat the oven until it reaches the temperature of 350 degrees F.

2. With a mixer at medium speed, beat margarine and sugar until they turn light and fluffy. Add egg white, vanilla and egg into the mixture. Slowly add cocoa and flour. Beat well. Pour the resulting mixture in a square pan (preferably 8-inch) coated with cooking spray.

3. Bean sweetener and cream cheese using a mixer at high speed. Add milk. Pour cream cheese on top of the chocolate mixture. Use the tip of the knife to swirl them together to create a marble-like effect.

4. Bake them at 350 degrees F for thirty minutes. Let it cool on a wire rack.

Low-Cholesterol Cinnamon-Flavored Streusel Crisps

Preparation Time: 20 minutes

Cooking Time: 20 minutes

Yield: 28 servings

Calories: 87

Ingredients:

- 1 package of refrigerated sugar cookie dough
- ¾ teaspoon of ground cinnamon
- ¼ cup of packed brown sugar (light)
- ¼ teaspoon of ground nutmeg
- ¼ cup of finely chopped pecans

Instructions:

1. Preheat oven until it reaches the temperature of 350 degrees F. Place the rack at the very center of the preheated oven.

2. Place the sugar cookie dough in a high-powered freezer for an hour. After an hour, transfer them in a cutting board. Cut them into 1/4 –inch slices which will yield to about 28-32 slices. Arrange them on a parchment paper-lined baking sheet.

3. Meanwhile, combine chopped oceans, cinnamon, nutmeg, and brown sugar in a small bowl to form a streusel. Top the cookies with ¾ teaspoon of streusel. Bake them in the preheated oven for twelve minutes.

4. Let it cool for 3 minutes before transferring them to a wire rack to fully cool down.

Lemon-Vanilla Berry Parfaits

Preparation Time: 10 minutes

Yield: 4 servings

Calories: 176

Ingredients:

- 1 cup of low-fat yogurt

- 2 tablespoons of honey

- 2 containers of vanilla pudding (fat-free)

- 1 lemon zest

- 2 tablespoons of lemon curd (bottled)

- Fresh mint leaves

- 1 tablespoon of lemon juice (fresh)

- ½ teaspoon of vanilla extract

- 3 cups of mixed berries (such as strawberries, raspberries and blueberries)

Instructions:

1. Whisk together the pudding, yogurt, vanilla extract and lemon curd in a small bowl. Set aside.

2. Mix lemon zest, lemon juice and honey in another mixing bowl. Stir well until fully

combined. Add in the mixed berries. Use a rubber spatula to gently stir to coat.

3. Assemble the parfaits in four glasses (preferably 8-ounce glasses). Scoop three tablespoons of the yogurt mixture in each glass. Top them with ¼ cup of mixed berries then another 3 tablespoons of the yogurt mixture then another ¼ cup of berries.

4. Garnish each parfait with fresh mint. Cover. Refrigerate for two hours. Enjoy.

Phase 7: Set Up Your Meal Plan

As was stated a while ago, the success of your TLC diet is going to depend on your ability to commit to the plan. A TLC Meal Plan can help you stay on track. Here's a sample meal plan to get you started.

The layout might be different from one person to another but it should look like this:

Monday

Breakfast: Spinach, Feta, and Tomato Omelet
Lunch: Orecchiette with Chickpeas and Broccoli Rabe
Dessert: Strawberry Shortcakes
Dinner: Garlic Chicken

Tuesday

Breakfast: Caramelized Onion, Parmesan Cheese and Arugula Omelet
Lunch: Lemon and Almond Crusted Fish with Spinach
Dessert: Lemon-Vanilla Berry Parfaits
Dinner: Chickpea Curry

Wednesday

Breakfast: Swiss Asparagus Omelet
Lunch: Tomato and Turkey Panini
Dessert: Cream Cheese Brownies
Dinner: Penne with Asparagus and Chicken

Thursday
Breakfast: Pasta Toss
Lunch: Slow-Cooked Pulled Pork BBQ
Dessert: Pretzel Turtles
Dinner: Black Beans and Rice

Friday
Breakfast: Spinach, Feta, and Tomato Omelet
Lunch: Honeyed Garlic Chicken
Dessert: Strawberry Shortcakes
Dinner: Chickpea Curry

Saturday
Breakfast: Buttermilk Pancakes
Lunch: Penne with Asparagus and Chicken
Dessert: Cream Cheese Brownies
Dinner: Tomato and Turkey Panini

Sunday
Breakfast: Apple-Cinnamon Granola Breakfast
Lunch: Lemon and Almond Crusted Fish with Spinach
Dessert: Cinnamon-Flavored Streusel Crisps
Dinner: Pulled Pork BBQ

You can mix and match the recommended meals to suit your budget. You could even add your own meals outside from the recommended recipes so as long as they are compatible with the goals of your TLC diet.

The point here is to commit yourself to the plan you have set yourself. This is because the diet will only work if you can control the portions of your meals and keep your daily intake below the maximum level of 2500 calories.

Conclusion

With all that is said and done, does the TLC diet work? The answer is yes. However, its success is completely dependent on the person using it: you.

Your ability to mentally prepare yourself for the plans and commit to it will make sure that your body gets the nutrients it needs while also burning through its stored fat. It will also help if you can be as realistic as possible while monitoring the progress in your diet.

If you implement the plan properly, you should see considerable changes occurring in your body. If you feel that you are ready to follow the requirements of this plan, it's best to get started as soon as possible.

Write a Review!

If you enjoyed this book, please take the time to share your thoughts and post a review.

Thank you and good luck!

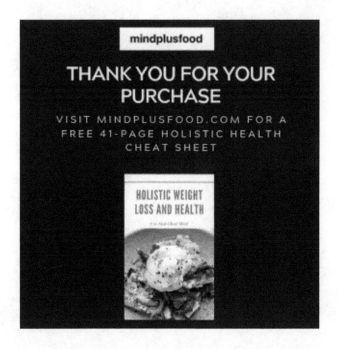

CPSIA information can be obtained
at www.ICGtesting.com
Printed in the USA
LVHW010410070121
675505LV00003B/403

9 781087 901879